Parkinson's disease

My story

by Diane Anglin

The first thing a person thinks of when they hear the words Parkinson's disease is trimmers. That is far from the truth. There are so many more symptoms than just a little trimmer.

There is stiffness, muscle spasms uncontrollable movements, it interferes with walking, hand movements. It effects every part of your body.

Chapter 1
The battle begins

I was diagnosed with Parkinson's disease at the age of 48. I am now 62. The battle has grown harder each year. It seems like each year it gets a little worse.

When I first found out I had Parkinson's disease I never dreamed it would be this devastating. I went from a healthy 48-year-old to a 62-year-old crippled.

Most of my days are spent writing on the computer, watching a movie on TV are just playing with my grandkids. Some days I spend just thinking about how things used to be before I had Parkinson's disease. Like walking and just doing my housework.

I am almost entirely dependent on my family. My hands don't work I can walk only a few feet I need assistance with just about everything I do.

The thing that really worries me is that there is no cure for this dreaded disease. There are medicines that help but the medicines can only do so much. In this book I will tell you how I made it this long.

Chapter 2
The family

Not only does the Parkinson's patients suffer but the family suffers as well. It is hard watching a loved one suffer and to see them fade away and become a different person. It is hard to tell your mother or father what they must do when you feel that they are the ones who should be telling you what to do it is like a role reversal.

The best thing a family can do for Parkinson's patients is to have knowledge of what Parkinson's disease is. You can find information about Parkinson's disease on the Internet, the Parkinson's foundation and through attending Parkinson's meetings both for the patients and the caregivers.

It is so hard to tell your mother grandmother whoever the patient is, to move their leg, knowing it is almost impossible for her to move her leg OR to eat when you know they have swallowing difficulties.

Chapter 3
The caregiver

The patient who has Parkinson's disease is the number one subject but we have to remember the caregiver. The caregiver is usually a spouse. The spouse usually takes over the role of caregiver at first because they love their spouse and think they can give them the best care. As the disease progresses the spouse finds it harder to take care of his loved one. The caregiver then becomes frustrated.

At this point the caregiver needs someone they can talk to they also need to ask for help. Whether you hire someone to come in two or three days a week to help or depend on family and friends to help either way caregivers need a break.

The caregiver has to make time for themselves. They need to get away from the patient at least an hour a day.

Chapter 4
Parkinson's patient

Having Parkinson's disease can be very depressing and some people even lose the desire to live but you can't think like that. There's always someone worse off than you. There will be anger, pity parties, fear of the unknown and fear of now. There will be all kinds of emotions. Some days you may be up others you may be down , remember that you have control over what you're thinking and what you allow your mind to think on.

If you allow your mind to think on bad things it will be harder to cope with your disease.

I found that to be positive and to think positive are the best tools the Parkinson's disease patient can use. To be negative hurts you and the people around you it is no benefit to your disease. To be positive gives you a better outlook on life. It motivates you to do things if it's only reading a book. Positive thinking that you can get better, that there are treatments.

I have always been a negative person and to think positive was very hard for me. It is something you have to work on every day, no matter what your disease is without being positive your life could be almost unbearable.

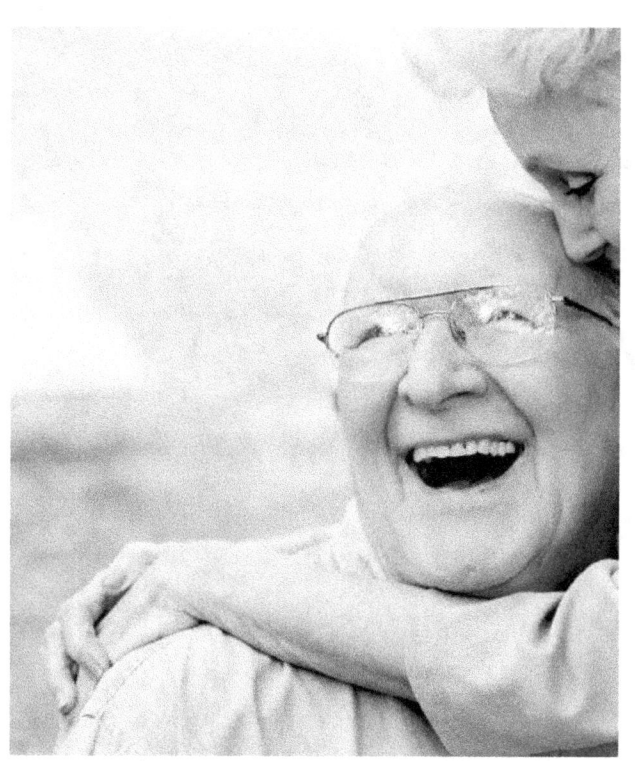

chapter 5
Caregiver

The caregiver needs as much help
as the patient, it is like having a
baby to take care of. At first
things might not seem very hard
but as the disease progresses it
gets harder to take care of the
Parkinson's patient as their needs
become more personal and
harder to deal with. The patient
often becomes impatient and
puts more demands on the
caregiver.

That is why it is so important for
the caregiver to attend
Parkinson's meetings so they can
learn how to cope with their
loved one. They can also interact
with other caregivers and share
experiences and exchange
information. It also gives the
caregiver a chance to get away
for a couple of hours. Getting out
of the house and away from the
patient for only a couple hours a
week can do wonders. The
caregiver is often overlooked by
others in having their needs met.
There should be a backup person

to care for the Parkinson's patient in case the caregiver is no longer able to care for their loved ones.

The caregiver also needs care. They need someone to relieve them if only a few hours a week from the stress of taking care of their loved one. Most say they don't need any help but they really do. The family needs to encourage the caregiver.

Chapter 6

Once I reached the point where I could no longer walk and it was very hard to move my hands I felt like giving up. I didn't want to get up in the morning I didn't want to face another day. The depression was as bad as the Parkinson's disease.

My doctor put me on an antidepressant and I began to feel a little better. I would talk myself out of getting into bad moods. I tried to focus on the good things in my life such as my family my grandchildren. I tried to stay positive. I would tell myself I will get better or maybe I don't have Parkinson's disease.

Some days I talked myself into believing I really didn't have Parkinson's disease. Too soon I was reminded that I do have Parkinson's disease and I needed to learn to cope with it.

Coping with PD was the hardest thing I have ever done. It is a part of my daily life, trying to cope. I always believed I had faith in God. If I had any faith I needed every ounce I could find. I would set in the same chair for hours what else is there for me to do? I had given up several times only to bounce back up again.

Parkinson's disease has stolen so much from me, my friends, my hobbies, my just going out to eat a meal with my husband. I find myself getting mad at God and asking why? I never got an answer and probably never will know the reason I have this disease.

Chapter 7
my faith in God

I became a Christian at the age of
13 and I knew the power of
prayer. Even though I had seen
God do so many miracles I
couldn't believe for my own
healing. It seems every time I
prayed things got worse.

Even though I was getting worse I
found that God did hear my
prayers, that he was there all the
time, even when I couldn't feel
his presence he was there,
guiding me, encouraging me.

Without my faith I could not
make it. Faith is the substance of
things hoped for the evidence of
things not yet seen. (John eight,
25.

To have faith in God we have to
have a spiritual mind. To have a
spiritual mind brings life and
peace. A carnal mind brings
death. I had to change the way I
think in order to get better. I had
to learn to trust God.

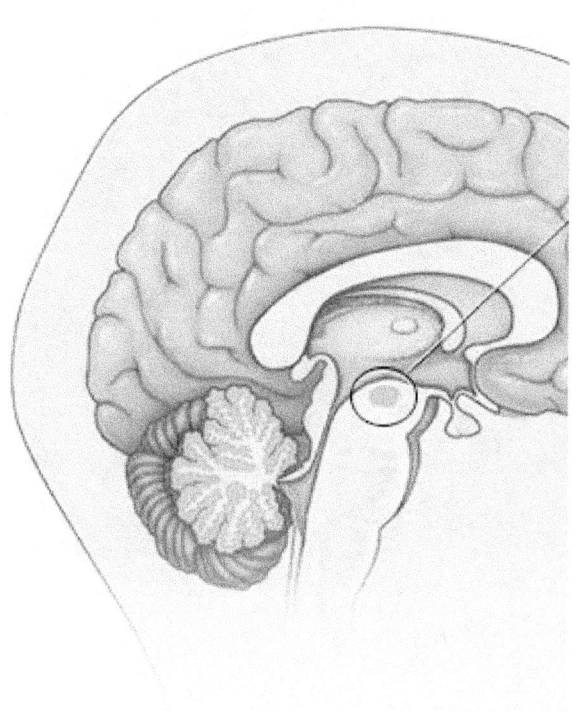

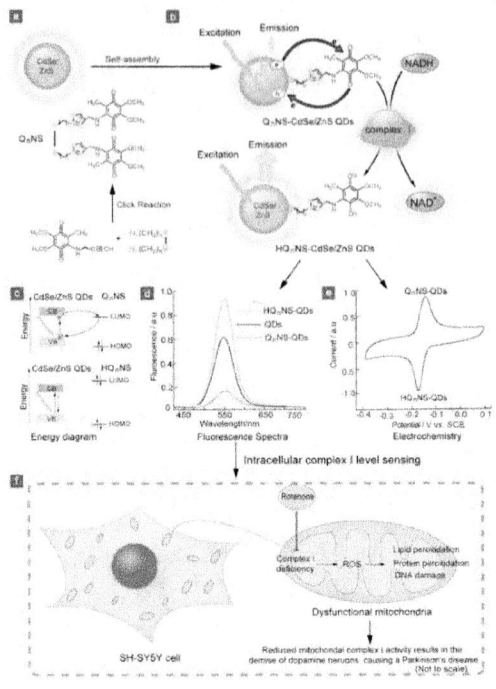

Chapter 8
Helping yourself

Getting in your car and going for a ride. Attending church, spending time with your grandkids and family

Watching movies that you like.

Talking to old friends.

If you can't get out of the house try sitting in a sunny place and just listen to the birds singing. Don't take for granted the things that you can do,

lose weight if you are overweight

try to move as often as possible.

Don't give up. A cure for
Parkinson's disease may be just
around the corner.

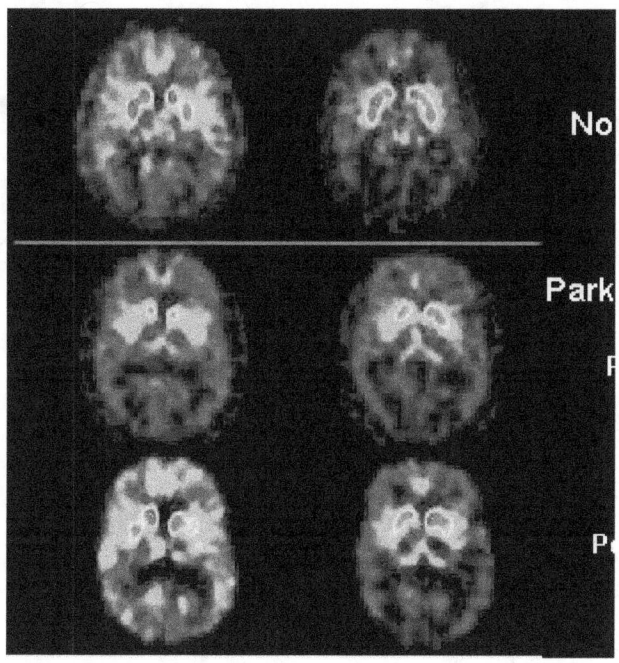

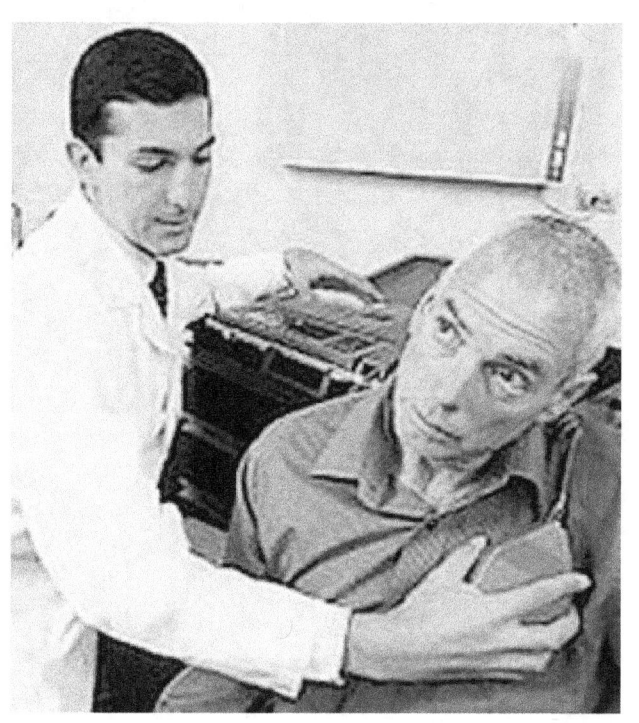

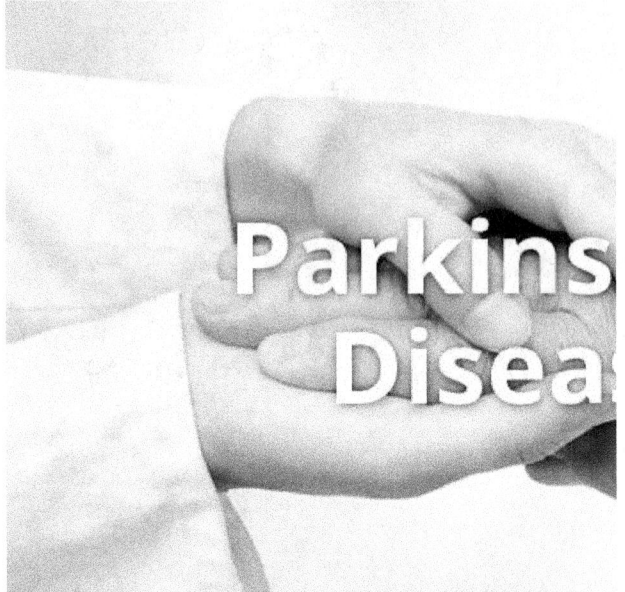

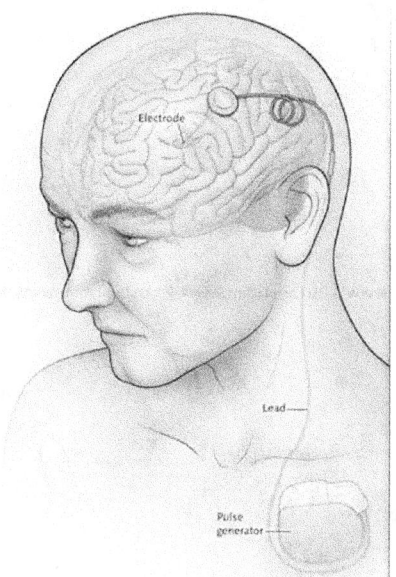